The Ultimate Keto Diet Cookbook

Enjoy Simple, Healthy and Savory Keto Recipes to Lose Weight Fast

Juliana Diaz

Table of Content

SMOOTHIES & BREAKFAST

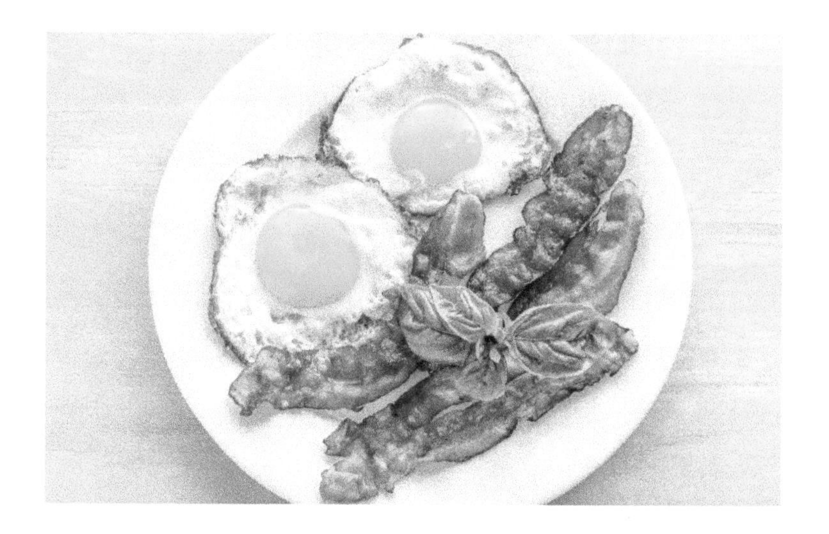

Chaffle with Sausage Gravy

Preparation Time: 5 minutes Cooking Time: 15 minutes Servings: 2

Ingredients:

- **¼ cup sausage, cooked**
- **3 tablespoons chicken broth**
- **2 teaspoons cream cheese**
- **2 tablespoons heavy whipping cream**
- **¼ teaspoon garlic powder**
- **Pepper to taste**
- **2 basic chaffles**

Directions:

1. **Add the sausage, broth, cream cheese, cream, garlic powder and pepper to a pan over medium heat.**

2. **Bring to a boil and then reduce heat.**

3. **Simmer for 10 minutes or until the sauce has thickened.**

4. **Pour the gravy on top of the basic chaffles**

5. **Serve.**

Nutrition:

Calories 212 Total Fat 17 g Saturated Fat 10 g Cholesterol 134 mg Sodium 350 mg Potassium 133 mg Total Carbohydrate 3 g Dietary Fiber 1 g Protein 11 g Total Sugars 1 g

Broccoli & Cheese Chaffle

Preparation Time: 5 minutes Cooking Time: 8 minutes Servings: 2

Ingredients:

- ¼ cup broccoli florets
- 1 egg, beaten
- 1 tablespoon almond flour
- ¼ teaspoon garlic powder
- ½ cup cheddar cheese

Directions:

1. Preheat your waffle maker.
2. Add the broccoli to the food processor.
3. Pulse until chopped.
4. Add to a bowl.
5. Stir in the egg and the rest of the ingredients.

6. **Mix well.**

7. **Pour half of the batter to the waffle maker.**

8. **Cover and cook for 4 minutes.**

9. **Repeat procedure to make the next chaffle.**

Nutrition: Calories 170 Total Fat 13 g Saturated Fat 7 g Cholesterol 112 mg Sodium 211 mg Potassium 94 mg Total Carbohydrate 2 g Dietary Fiber 1 g Protein 11 g Total Sugars 1 g

Creamy Chicken Mushrooms

Preparation Time: 10 minutes

Cooking Time: 30 minutes Serve: 4

Ingredients:

- 2 lbs chicken breasts, halved
- 1/4 cup sun-dried tomatoes
- 7.5 oz mushrooms, sliced
- ½ cup mayonnaise
- 1 tsp salt

Directions:

1. Preheat the oven to 400 F.
2. Place chicken breasts into the greased baking dish and top with sun-dried tomatoes, mushrooms, mayonnaise, and salt. Mix well.
3. Bake in the oven for 30 minutes.
4. Serve and enjoy.

Nutritional Value (Amount per Serving):

Calories 561

Fat 27 g

Carbohydrates 10 g

Sugar 4 g

Protein 68 g

Cholesterol 210 mg

Pumpkin & Pecan Chaffle

Preparation Time: 5 minutes Cooking Time: 10 minutes Servings: 2

Ingredients:

- 1 egg, beaten
- ½ cup mozzarella cheese, grated
- ½ teaspoon pumpkin spice
- 1 tablespoon pureed pumpkin
- 2 tablespoons almond flour
- 1 teaspoon sweetener
- 2 tablespoons pecans, chopped

Directions:

1. Turn on the waffle maker.
2. Beat the egg in a bowl.
3. Stir in the rest of the ingredients.
4. Pour half of the mixture into the device.
5. Seal the lid.

6. **Cook for 5 minutes.**
7. **Remove the chaffle carefully.**
8. **Repeat the steps to make the second chaffle.**

Nutrition: Calories 210 Total Fat 17 g Saturated Fat 10 g Cholesterol 110
mg Sodium 250 mg Potassium 570 mg Total Carbohydrate 4.6 g Dietary Fiber 1.7 g Protein 11 g Total Sugars 2 g

Apple Pie Chaffles

Preparation Time: 10 minutes Cooking Time: 14 minutes Servings: 2

Ingredients:

- ½ cup finely grated mozzarella cheese
- 1 egg, beaten
- ¼ tsp apple pie spice
- 4 butter slices for serving

Directions:

1. Preheat the waffle iron.
2. Open the iron, pour in half of the mozzarella cheese in the iron, top with half of the egg, and sprinkle with half of the apple pie spice.
3. Close the iron and cook until crispy, 6 to 7 minutes.
4. Remove the chaffle onto a plate and set aside.
5. Make the second chaffle with the remaining ingredients.

6. **Allow cooling and serve after.**

Nutrition: Calories 146; Fats 14.73g; Carbs 0.9g; Net Carbs 0.7g; Protein 3.07g

Spicy Shrimp and Chaffles

Preparation Time: 15 minutes
Cooking Time: 31 minutes Servings: 4

Ingredients:
For the shrimp:

- 1 tbsp olive oil
- 1 lb jumbo shrimp, peeled and deveined
- 1 tbsp Creole seasoning
- Salt to taste
- 2 tbsp hot sauce
- 3 tbsp butter
- 2 tbsp chopped fresh scallions to garnish

For the chaffles:

- 2 eggs, beaten
- 1 cup finely grated Monterey Jack cheese

Directions:

For the shrimp:

1. Heat the olive oil in a medium skillet over medium heat.

2. Season the shrimp with the Creole seasoning and salt. Cook in the oil until pink and opaque on both sides, 2

   minutes.

3. Pour in the hot sauce and butter. Mix well until the shrimp is adequately coated in the sauce, 1 minute.

4. Turn the heat off and set aside.

For the chaffles:

2. Preheat the waffle iron.

3. In a medium bowl, mix the eggs and Monterey Jack cheese.

4. Open the iron and add a quarter of the mixture. Close and cook until crispy, 7 minutes.

5. Transfer the chaffle to a plate and make 3 more chaffles in the same manner.

6. Cut the chaffles into quarters and place

on a plate.

7. **Top with the shrimp and garnish with the scallions.**

8. **Serve warm.**

Nutrition: Calories 342 Fats 19.75g Carbs 2.8g Net Carbs 2.3g Protein 36.01g

Keto Reuben Chaffles

Preparation Time: 15 minutes Cooking Time: 28 minutes Servings: 4

Ingredients:

For the chaffles:

- 2 eggs, beaten
- 1 cup finely grated Swiss cheese
- 2 tsp caraway seeds
- 1/8 tsp salt
- ½ tsp baking powder

For the sauce:

- 2 tbsp sugar-free ketchup
- 3 tbsp mayonnaise
- 1 tbsp dill relish
- 1 tsp hot sauce

For the filling:

- 6 oz pastrami
- 2 Swiss cheese slices
- ¼ cup pickled radishes

Directions:

For the chaffles:

1. **Preheat the waffle iron.**

2. **In a medium bowl, mix the eggs, Swiss cheese, caraway seeds, salt, and baking powder.**

3. **Open the iron and add a quarter of the mixture. Close and cook until crispy, 7 minutes.**
4. **Transfer the chaffle to a plate and make 3 more chaffles in the same manner.**

For the sauce:

1. **In another bowl, mix the ketchup, mayonnaise, dill relish, and hot sauce.**

2. **To assemble:**

3. **Divide on two chaffles; the sauce, the pastrami, Swiss cheese slices, and pickled radishes.**

4. **Cover with the other chaffles, divide the sandwich in halves and serve.**

Nutrition: Calories 316 Fats 21.78g Carbs 6.52g Net Carbs 5.42g Protein 23.56g

Stuffed Jalapenos

Preparation Time: 10 minutes Cooking Time: 15 minutes

Serve: 12

Ingredients:

- 1/2 cup chicken, cooked and shredded
- 6 jalapenos, halved
- 3 tbsp green onion, sliced
- 1/4 cup cheddar cheese, shredded
- 1/2 tsp dried basil
- 1/4 tsp garlic powder
- 3 oz cream cheese
- 1/2 tsp dried oregano
- 1/4 tsp salt

Directions:

- Preheat the oven to 390 F.
- Mix all ingredients in a bowl except jalapenos.
- Stuff chicken mixture into each jalapeno halved and place on a baking tray.
- Bake for 25 minutes.
- Serve and enjoy.

Nutritional Value (Amount per Serving):

Calories 106

Fat 9 g

Carbohydrates 2 g

Sugar 1 g

Protein 7 g

Cholesterol 35 mg

PORK, BEEF & LAMB RECIPES

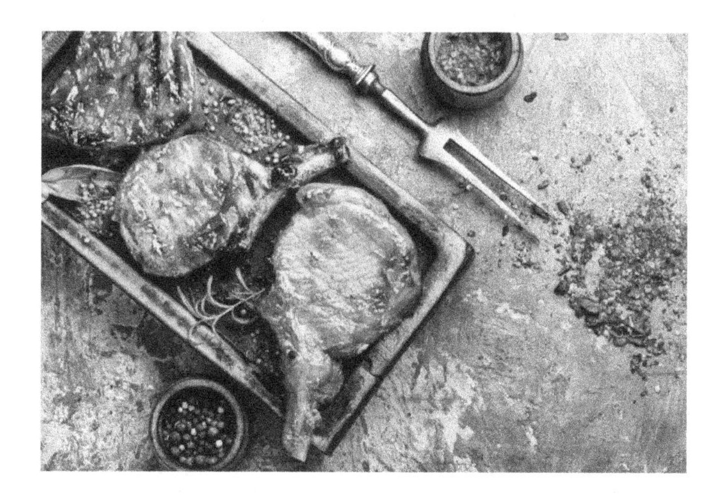

Pork Egg Roll Bowl

Preparation Time: 10 minutes Cooking Time: 10 minutes Serve: 6

Ingredients:

- 1 lb ground pork
- 3 tbsp soy sauce
- 1 tbsp sesame oil
- 1/2 onion, sliced
- 1 medium cabbage head, sliced
- 2 tbsp green onion, chopped
- 2 tbsp chicken broth
- 1 tsp ground ginger
- 2 garlic cloves, minced
- Pepper
- Salt

Directions:

1. Brown meat in a pan over medium heat.
2. Add oil and onion to the pan with meat. Mix well and cook over medium heat.
3. In a small bowl, mix together soy sauce, ginger, and garlic.
4. Add soy sauce mixture to the pan.

5. Add cabbage to the pan and toss to coat.
6. Add broth to the pan and mix well.
7. Cook over medium heat for 3 minutes.
8. Season with pepper and salt.
9. Garnish with green onion and serve. **Nutritional Value (Amount per Serving):** Calories 171

Fat 5 g

Carbohydrates 10 g

Sugar 5 g

Protein 23 g

Cholesterol 56 mg

Lemon Pepper Pork Tenderloin

Preparation Time: 10 minutes Cooking Time: 25 minutes Serve: 4

Ingredients:

- 1 lb pork tenderloin
- 3/4 tsp lemon pepper
- 1 1/2 tsp dried oregano
- 1 tbsp olive oil
- 4 tbsp feta cheese, crumbled
- 2 1/2 tbsp olive tapenade

Directions:

1. Add pork, oil, lemon pepper, and oregano in a zip-lock bag. Seal bag and rub well and place in a refrigerator for 2 hours.
2. Remove pork from zip-lock bag.
3. Using a sharp knife make lengthwise cut through the center of the tenderloin.
4. Spread olive tapenade on half tenderloin and sprinkle with crumbled cheese.
5. Fold another half of meat over to the original shape of tenderloin.
6. Close pork tenderloin with twine at 2- inch intervals.
7. Grill for 20 minutes. Turn tenderloin during grilling.
8. Sliced and serve.

Nutritional Value (Amount per Serving):

Calories 215

Fat 10 g

Carbohydrates 1 g

Sugar 1 g

Protein 31 g

Cholesterol 90 mg

SEAFOOD & FISH RECIPES

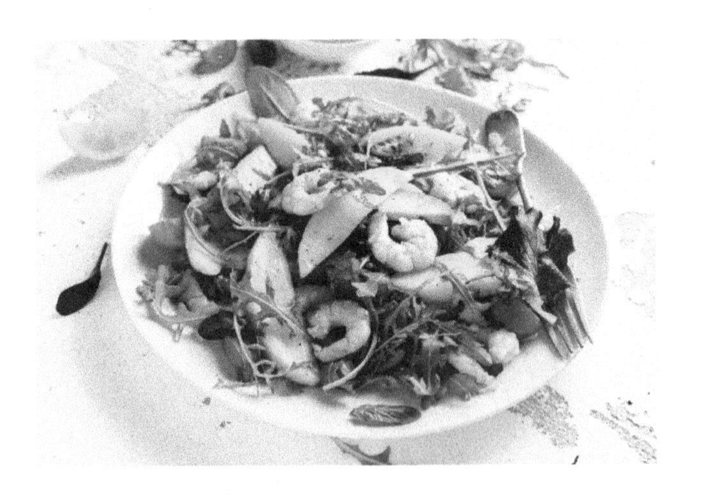

Grilled Salmon

Preparation Time: 10 minutes Cooking Time: 25 minutes

Serve: 4

Ingredients:

- 4 salmon fillets
- 1 tsp dried rosemary
- 3 garlic cloves, minced
- 1/4 tsp pepper
- 1 tsp salt

Directions:

1. In a bowl, mix together rosemary, garlic, pepper, and salt.
2. Add salmon fillets in a bowl and coat well and let sit for 15 minutes.
3. Preheat the grill.
4. Place marinated salmon fillets on hot grill and cook for 10-12 minutes.
5. Serve and enjoy.

Nutritional Value (Amount per Serving):

Calories 240

Fat 11 g

Carbohydrates 1 g

Sugar 0 g

Protein 34 g

Cholesterol 78 mg

MEATLESS MEALS

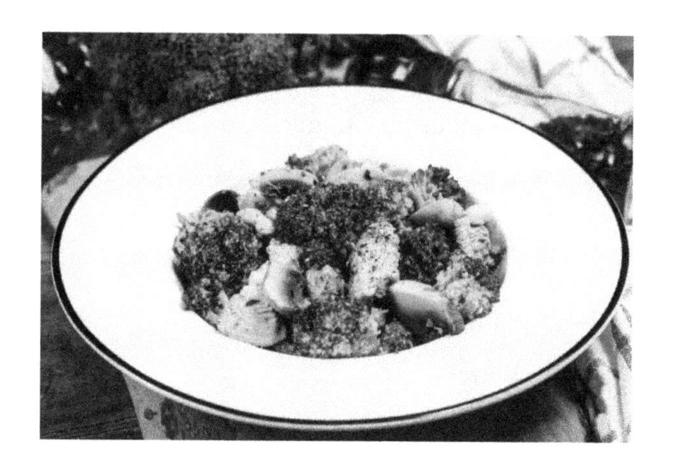

Creamy Cabbage

Preparation Time: 10 minutes Cooking Time: 15 minutes

Serve: 4

Ingredients:

- 1/2 cabbage head, shredded
- 3 garlic cloves, chopped
- 1 onion, sliced
- 1 bell pepper, cut into strips
- 2 tbsp butter
- 3 oz cream cheese
- ¼ tsp onion powder
- ¼ tsp garlic powder
- 1/2 tsp pepper
- 1 tsp kosher salt

Directions:

1. Melt butter in a saucepan over medium heat.
2. Add garlic and onion and sauté for 5 minutes.
3. Add cabbage and bell pepper and cook for 5 minutes.
4. Add remaining ingredients and stir well.
5. Serve and enjoy.

Nutritional Value (Amount per Serving):

Calories 170

Fat 13 g

Carbohydrates 12 g

Sugar 5 g

Protein 3 g

Cholesterol 40 mg

SOUPS, STEWS & SALADS

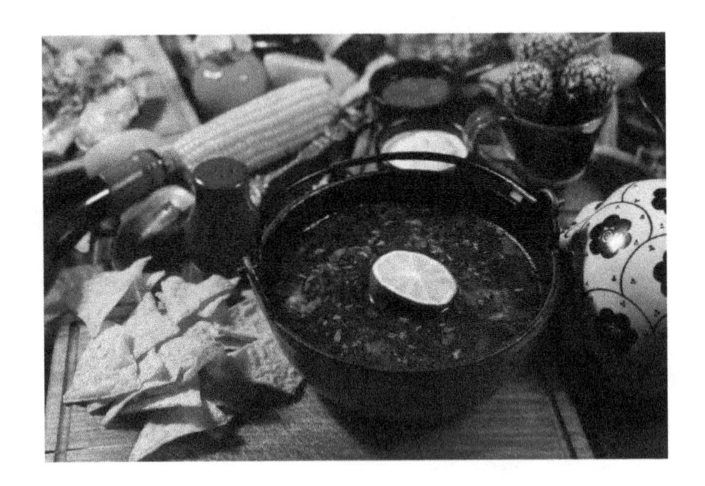

Ginger Carrot Soup

Preparation Time: 10 minutes Cooking Time: 10 minutes

Serve: 4

Ingredients:

- 4 carrots, peeled and chopped
- 1 tsp turmeric powder
- 3 cups vegetable stock
- 2 tsp coconut oil
- 3 garlic cloves, minced
- 1 onion, chopped
- 1 parsnip, peeled and chopped
- 1 tbsp fresh lemon juice
- 1/4 tsp cayenne pepper
- 1/2 tbsp ginger, grated

Directions:

1. Preheat the oven to 350 F.
2. Add carrots, garlic, onion, parsnip, coconut oil, and cayenne pepper in a bowl and toss well.
3. Spread bowl mixture on baking tray and roast in oven for 15 minutes.
4. Transfer roasted veggie in blender along with ginger, lemon juice, and stock into the blender and blend until smooth.
5. Serve and enjoy.

Nutritional Value (Amount per Serving):

Calories 72

Fat 4 g

Carbohydrates 11 g

Sugar 5 g

Protein 1 g

Cholesterol 0 mg

Cheese Mushroom Shrimp Soup

Preparation Time: 10 minutes Cooking Time: 15 minutes Serve: 8

Ingredients:

- 24 oz shrimp, cooked
- 8 oz cheddar cheese, shredded
- ½ cup butter
- 1 cup heavy cream
- 32 oz vegetable stock
- 2 cups mushrooms, sliced
- Pepper
- Salt

Directions:

1. Add stock and mushrooms to a large pot. Bring to boil.
2. Turn heat to medium and add cheese, heavy cream, and butter and stir until cheese is melted.
3. Add shrimp. Stir well and cook for 2 minutes more.
4. Serve and enjoy.

Nutritional Value (Amount per Serving):

Calories 390

Fat 28 g

Carbohydrates 3 g

Sugar 0.8 g

Protein 30 g

Cholesterol 17

mg

BRUNCH & DINNER

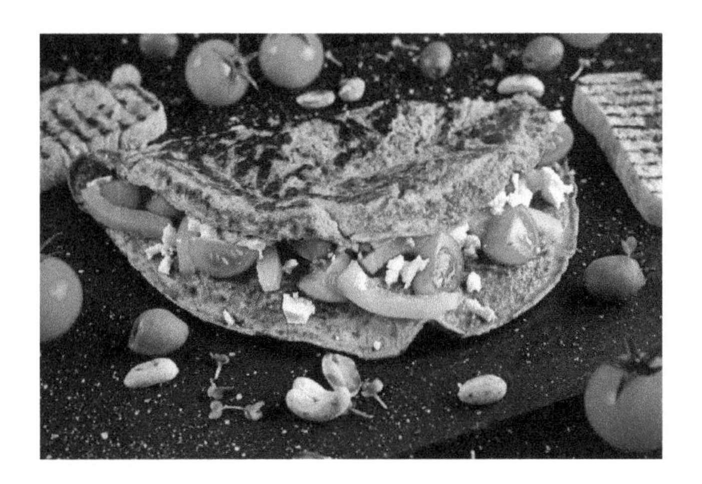

Coconut Kale Muffins

Preparation Time: 10 minutes Cooking Time: 30 minutes

Serve: 8

Ingredients:

- 6 eggs
- 1/2 cup unsweetened coconut milk
- 1 cup kale, chopped
- ¼ tsp garlic powder
- ¼ tsp paprika
- 1/4 cup green onion, chopped
- Pepper
- Salt

Directions:

1. Preheat the oven to 350 F.
2. Add all ingredients into the bowl and whisk well.
3. Pour mixture into the greased muffin tray and bake in oven for 30 minutes.
4. Serve and enjoy.

Nutritional Value (Amount per Serving):

Calories 92

Fat 7 g

Carbohydrates 2 g

Sugar 0.8 g

Protein 5 g

Cholesterol 140 mg

DESSERTS & DRINKS

Protein Peanut Butter Ice Cream

Preparation Time: 5 minutes Cooking Time: 5 minutes

Serve: 2

Ingredients:

- 5 drops liquid stevia
- 2 tbsp heavy cream
- 2 tbsp peanut butter
- 2 tbsp protein powder
- ¾ cup cottage cheese

Directions:

1. Add all ingredients into the blender and blend until smooth.
2. Pour blended mixture into the container and place in refrigerator for 30 minutes.
3. Serve chilled and enjoy.

Nutritional Value (Amount per Serving):

Calories 222

Fat 15 g

Carbohydrates 7 g

Sugar 2 g

Protein 16 g

Cholesterol 27 mg

BREAKFAST RECIPES

Mini Bacon Guacamole Cups

Serves: 4

Prep Time: 40 mins

Ingredients

- 1 ripe avocado
- 9 bacon slices, 6 slices halved, and 3 slices quartered
- 2 tablespoons onion, minced
- Kosher salt and black pepper, to taste
- 1 small jalapeno, seeded and minced

Directions

1. Preheat the oven to 4000F and turn 4 mini-muffin pans upside down on a baking sheet.
2. Spray the tops of the overturned muffin tins and place the quarter of the slice on top.
3. Wrap the sides of the mini-muffin pans with the longer portions of bacon and secure with a toothpick.
4. Bake for about 25 minutes and remove carefully from the mini muffin cups.

5. Meanwhile, mash avocado with a fork in a medium bowl and stir in the jalapeno, onions, salt and black pepper.
6. Put the guacamole in the bacon cups and serve warm.

Nutrition Amount per serving

Calories 337

Total Fat 27.7g 36%

Saturated Fat 7.9g 40% Cholesterol 47mg 16%

Sodium 991mg 43%

Total Carbohydrate 5.6g 2% Dietary Fiber 3.6g

13% Total Sugars 0.6g

Protein 16.9g

Breakfast Bacon Muffins

Serves: 6

Prep Time: 30 mins

Ingredients

- 1 cup bacon bits
- 3 cups almond flour, organic
- ½ cup ghee, melted
- 1 teaspoon baking soda
- 4 eggs

Directions

1. Preheat the oven to 3500F and line muffin tins with muffin liners.
2. Melt ghee in a bowl and stir in the almond flour and baking soda.
3. Mix well and add the bacon bits and eggs.
4. Divide the mixture into the muffin tins and transfer into the oven.
5. Bake for about 20 minutes and remove from the oven to serve.

Nutrition Amount per serving

Calories 485

Total Fat 49.8g 64% Saturated Fat 37.3g 186% Cholesterol

156mg 52%

Sodium 343mg 15%

Total Carbohydrate 6.9g 3% Dietary Fiber 2.6g 9%

Total Sugars 4.2g Protein 7.7g

APPETIZERS & DESSERTS

Garlicky Green Beans Stir Fry

Serves: 4

Prep Time: 25 mins

Ingredients

- 2 tablespoons peanut oil
- 1 pound fresh green beans
- 2 tablespoons garlic, chopped
- Salt and red chili pepper, to taste
- ½ yellow onion, slivered

Directions

1. Heat peanut oil in a wok over high heat and add garlic and onions.
2. Sauté for about 4 minutes add beans, salt and red chili pepper.
3. Sauté for about 3 minutes and add a little water.
4. Cover with lid and cook on low heat for about 5 minutes.
5. Dish out into a bowl and serve hot.

Nutrition Amount per serving

Calories 107 Total Fat 6.9g 9%

Saturated Fat 1.2g 6% Cholesterol 0mg 0%

Sodium 8mg 0%

Total Carbohydrate 10.9g 4% Dietary Fiber 4.3g 15%

Total Sugars 2.3g Protein 2.5g

PORK AND BEEF RECIPES

Zesty Pork Chops

Serves: 4

Prep Time: 50 mins

Ingredients

- 4 tablespoons butter
- 3 tablespoons lemon juice
- 4 pork chops, bone-in
- 2 tablespoons low carb flour mix
- 1 cup picante sauce

Directions

1. Coat the pork chops with low carb flour mix.
2. Mix picante sauce and lemon juice in a bowl.
3. Heat oil in a skillet on medium heat and add the chops and picante mixture.
4. Cook covered for about 35 minutes and dish out to serve hot.

Nutrition Amount per serving

Calories 398

Total Fat 33.4g 43% Saturated Fat 15g 75%

Cholesterol 99mg 33%

Sodium 441mg 19%

Total Carbohydrate 4g 1% Dietary Fiber 0.7g 3%

Total Sugars 2.1g

Protein 19.7g

SEAFOOD RECIPES

Broccoli and Cheese

Serves: 4

Prep Time: 20 mins

Ingredients

- 5½ oz. cheddar cheese, shredded
- 23 oz. broccoli, chopped
- 2 oz. butter
- Salt and black pepper, to taste
- 4 tablespoons sour cream

Directions

1. Heat butter in a large skillet over medium high heat and add broccoli, salt and black pepper.
2. Cook for about 5 minutes and stir in the sour cream and cheddar cheese.
3. Cover with lid and cook for about 8 minutes on medium low heat.
4. Dish out to a bowl and serve hot.

Nutrition Amount per serving

Calories 340

Total Fat 27.5g 35% Saturated Fat 17.1g 85%

Cholesterol 77mg 26%

Sodium 384mg 17%

Total Carbohydrate 11.9g 4% Dietary Fiber 4.3g 15%

Total Sugars 3g Protein 14.8g

CHICKEN AND POULTRY RECIPES

Caprese Chicken

Serves: 4

Prep Time: 30 mins

Ingredients

- 1 pound chicken breasts, boneless and skinless
- ¼ cup balsamic vinegar
- 1 tablespoon extra-virgin olive oil
- Kosher salt and black pepper, to taste
- 4 mozzarella cheese slices

Directions

1. Season the chicken with salt and black pepper.
2. Heat olive oil in a skillet over medium heat and cook chicken for about 5 minutes on each side.
3. Stir in the balsamic vinegar and cook for about 2 minutes.
4. Add mozzarella cheese slices and cook for about 2 minutes until melted.
5. Dish out in a plate and serve hot.

Nutrition Amount per serving

Calories 329

Total Fat 16.9g 22% Saturated Fat 5.8g 29% Cholesterol 116mg 39%

Sodium 268mg 12%

Total Carbohydrate 1.1g 0%

Dietary Fiber 0g 0%

Total Sugars 0.1g

Protein 40.8g

Roasted Chicken with Herbed Butter

Serves: 6

Prep Time: 30 mins

Ingredients

- 1 tablespoon garlic paste
- 6 chicken legs
- 4 cups water
- Salt, to taste
- 4 tablespoons herbed butter

Directions

1. Season the chicken legs with salt and mix with garlic paste.
2. Put a rack in an electric pressure cooker and add water.
3. Place the marinated pieces of chicken on the rack and lock the lid.
4. Cook on high pressure for about 15 minutes.
5. Naturally release the pressure and dish out in a platter.
6. Spread herbed butter on the chicken legs and serve.

Nutrition Amount per serving

Calories 304

Total Fat 12.7g 16% Saturated Fat 3.8g 19% Cholesterol 137mg 46%

Sodium 177mg 8%

Total Carbohydrate 0.7g 0% Dietary Fiber 0g 0%

Total Sugars 0.1g

Protein 44g

Chicken Enchiladas

Serves: 2

Prep Time: 25 mins

Ingredients

- 2 ounces chicken, shredded
- ½ tablespoon olive oil
- 2 ounces shiitake mushrooms, chopped
- Sea salt and black pepper, to taste
- ½ teaspoon apple cider vinegar

Directions

1. Heat olive oil in a skillet and add mushrooms.
2. Sauté for about 30 seconds and stir in chicken.
3. Cook for about 2 minutes and pour in apple cider vinegar.
4. Season with sea salt and black pepper and cover the lid.
5. Cook for about 20 minutes on medium low heat.
6. Dish out and serve hot.

Nutrition Amount per serving

Calories 88

Total Fat 4.4g 6% Saturated Fat 0.8g 4%

Cholesterol 22mg 7%

Sodium 86mg 4%

Total Carbohydrate 3.9g 1%

Dietary Fiber 0.6g 2%

Total Sugars 1g

Protein 8.7g

Turkey Balls

Serves: 6

Prep Time: 35 mins

Ingredients

- 1 cup broccoli, chopped
- 1 pound turkey, boiled and chopped
- 2 teaspoons ginger-garlic paste
- Salt and lemon pepper seasoning, to taste
- ½ cup olive oil

Directions

1. Preheat the oven to 3600F and grease a baking tray.
2. Mix together turkey, olive oil, broccoli, ginger-garlic paste, salt and lemon pepper seasoning in a bowl.
3. Make small balls out of this mixture and arrange on the baking tray.
4. Transfer to the oven and bake for about 20 minutes.
5. Remove from the oven and serve with the dip of your choice.

Nutrition Amount per serving

Calories 275

Total Fat 20.1g 26%

Saturated Fat 3g 15%

Cholesterol 58mg 19%

Sodium 53mg 2%

Total Carbohydrate 1.5g 1% Dietary Fiber 0.4g 1%

Total Sugars 0.3g

Protein 22.4g

Air Fried Chicken

Serves: 2

Prep Time: 20 mins

Ingredients

- 1 tablespoon olive oil
- 4 skinless, boneless chicken tenderloins
- 1 egg
- Salt and black pepper, to taste
- ½ teaspoon turmeric powder

Directions

1. Preheat the air fryer to 3700F and coat the fryer basket with olive oil.
2. Beat the egg and dip the chicken tenderloins in it.
3. Mix together turmeric powder, salt and black pepper in a bowl and dredge chicken tenderloins.
4. Arrange the chicken tenderloins in the fryer basket and cook for about 10 minutes.
5. Dish out on a platter and serve with salsa.

Nutrition Amount per serving

Calories 304

Total Fat 15.2g 20% Saturated Fat 4g 20%

Cholesterol 179mg 60%

Sodium 91mg 4%

Total Carbohydrate 0.6g 0% Dietary Fiber 0.1g 0%

Total Sugars 0.2g Protein 40.3g

BREAKFAST RECIPES

Grain-free

Overnight Oats

Total Time: 10 minutes Serves: 1

Ingredients:

- 2/3 cup unsweetened coconut milk
- 2 tsp chia seeds
- 2 tbsp vanilla protein powder
- ½ tbsp coconut flour
- 3 tbsp hemp hearts

Directions:

1. Add all ingredients into the glass jar and stir to combine.
2. Close jar with lid and place in refrigerator for overnight.
3. Top with fresh berries and serve.

Nutritional Value (Amount per Serving): Calories 378; Fat 22.5 g; Carbohydrates 15 g; Sugar 1.5 g; Protein 27 g; Cholesterol 0mg;

Breakfast Granola

Total Time: 30 minutes Serves: 15

Ingredients:

- 1 tsp ground ginger
- 1 tsp ground cinnamon
- ¼ cups coconut oil, melted
- 1 cup walnuts, chopped
- 2/3 cup pumpkin seeds
- 2/3 cup sunflower seeds
- ½ cup flaxseeds
- 3 cups desiccated coconut

Directions:

1. Add all ingredients into the large bowl and toss well.
2. Spread granola mixture on a baking tray and bake at 350 F/ 180 C for 20 minutes. Turn granola mixture with a spoon after every 3 minutes.
3. Allow to cool completely and serve.

Nutritional Value (Amount per Serving): Calories 208; Fat 17 g; Carbohydrates 11.4 g; Sugar 5.8 g; Protein 4.1 g; Cholesterol 0 mg;

LUNCH RECIPES

Turnip Salad

Total Time: 10 minutes Serves: 4

Ingredients:

- 4 white turnips, spiralized
- 1 lemon juice
- 4 dill sprigs, chopped
- 2 tbsp olive oil
- 1 1/2 tsp salt

Directions:

1. Season spiralized turnip with salt and gently massage with hands.
2. Add lemon juice and dill. Season with pepper and salt.
3. Drizzle with olive oil and combine everything well.
4. Serve immediately and enjoy.

Nutritional Value (Amount per Serving): Calories 49; Fat 1.1 g; Carbohydrates 9 g;

Sugar 5.2 g; Protein 1.4 g; Cholesterol 0 mg;

Roasted Almond Broccoli

Total Time: 25 minutes Serves: 4

Ingredients:

- 1 1/2 lbs broccoli florets
- 3 tbsp olive oil
- 1 tbsp fresh lemon juice
- 3 tbsp slivered almonds, toasted
- 2 garlic cloves, sliced
- 1/4 tsp pepper
- 1/4 tsp salt

Directions:

1. Preheat the oven to 425 F/ 218 C.
2. Spray baking dish with cooking spray.
3. Add broccoli, pepper, salt, garlic, and oil in large bowl and toss well.
4. Spread broccoli on the prepared baking dish and roast in preheated oven for 20 minutes.
5. Add lemon juice and almonds over broccoli and toss well.
6. Serve and enjoy.

Nutritional Value (Amount per Serving):

Calories 177; Fat 13.3 g; Carbohydrates 12.9 g; Sugar 3.2 g; Protein 5.8 g; Cholesterol 0 mg;

DINNER RECIPES

Cauliflower Couscous

Total Time: 25 minutes Serves: 4

Ingredients:

- 1 head cauliflower, cut into florets
- 14 black olives
- 1 garlic cloves, chopped
- 14 oz can artichokes
- 2 tbsp olive oil
- 1/4 cup parsley, chopped
- 1 lemon juice
- 1/2 tsp pepper
- 1/2 tsp salt

Directions:

1. Preheat the oven to 400 F/ 200 C.
2. Add cauliflower florets into the food processor and process until it looks like rice.
3. Spread cauliflower rice on a baking tray and drizzle with olive oil. Bake in preheated oven for 12 minutes.
4. In a bowl, mix together garlic, lemon juice, artichokes, parsley, and olives.
5. Add cauliflower to the bowl and stir well. Season with pepper and salt.
6. Serve and enjoy.

Nutritional Value (Amount per Serving): Calories 116; Fat 8.8 g; Carbohydrates 8.4 g; Sugar 3.3 g; Protein 3.3 g; Cholesterol 0 mg

Basil Tomato Soup

Total Time: 20 minutes Serves: 6

Ingredients:

- 28 oz can tomatoes
- ¼ cup basil pesto
- ¼ tsp dried basil leaves
- 1 tsp apple cider vinegar
- 2 tbsp erythritol
- ¼ tsp garlic powder
- ½ tsp onion powder
- 2 cups water
- 1 ½ tsp kosher salt

Directions:

1. Add tomatoes, garlic powder, onion powder, water, and salt in a saucepan.
2. Bring to boil over medium heat. Reduce heat and simmer for 2 minutes.
3. Remove saucepan from heat and puree the soup using a blender until smooth.
4. Stir in pesto, dried basil, vinegar, and erythritol.
5. Stir well and serve warm.

Nutritional Value (Amount per Serving): Calories 30; Fat 0 g; Carbohydrates 12.1 g;

Sugar 9.6 g; Protein 1.3 g; Cholesterol 0 mg;

DESSERT RECIPES

Quick Chocó Brownie

Total Time: 10 minutes Serves: 1

Ingredients:

- 1/4 cup almond milk
- 1 tbsp cocoa powder
- 1 scoop chocolate protein powder
- 1/2 tsp baking powder

Directions:

In a microwave-safe mug blend together baking powder, protein powder, and cocoa.

1. Add almond milk in a mug and stir well.
2. Place mug in microwave and microwave for 30 seconds.
3. Serve and enjoy.

Nutritional Value (Amount per Serving): Calories 207; Fat 15.8 g; Carbohydrates 9.5 g; Sugar 3.1 g; Protein 12.4 g; Cholesterol 20 mg;

BREAKFAST RECIPES

Sausage Patties

No traditional breakfast would be complete without sausage patties. Packed with protein, these would be wonderful before your morning run.

Total Prep & Cooking Time: 20 minutes Level: Beginner

Makes: 4 Patties

Protein: 25 grams Net Carbs: 5.2 grams Fat: 9 grams

Sugar: 1 gram

Calories: 272

What you need:

- 1/3 tsp onion powder
- 3/4 lb. ground pork
- 1/3 tsp salt
- 4 3/4 oz. mushrooms, chopped
- 1/3 tsp garlic powder
- 4 oz. kale, thinly sliced
- 1/8 tsp ground ginger
- 2 tbs coconut oil, separated
- 1/8 tsp nutmeg
- 2 garlic cloves, minced
- 1/4 tsp fennel seeds

Steps:

1. Melt 1 tablespoon of coconut oil in a skillet.
2. Put in the mushrooms, minced garlic and kale and stir fry for approximately 5 minutes and remove from heat.
3. In a dish, combine the ground pork, cooked vegetables, onion powder, garlic powder, nutmeg, and fennel seeds.
4. Divide into 4 sections and create patties by hand.
5. In the same skillet, pour a tablespoon of coconut oil and heat.
6. Fry the patties for approximately 2 minutes and turn over to brown the other side. Flip over as necessary to fully cook the meat in the middle of the patties.
7. Serve immediately and enjoy.

Variation Tip:

You can choose to mix up the recipe using different meat or vegetables such as ground turkey or beef and spinach or bell peppers.

LUNCH RECIPES

Spicy Cauliflower Turkey

This moist dish will keep you satisfied throughout the day and have you coming back for seconds at dinnertime.

Total Prep & Cooking Time: 25 minutes Level: Beginner

Makes: 4 Helpings

Protein: 23 grams Net Carbs: 4.4 grams

Fat: 24 grams

Sugar: 0 grams

Calories: 310

What you need:

- 3/4 tsp salt
- 12 oz. ground turkey
- 3/4 tbs mustard
- 1 2/3 cups cauliflower
- 3/4 tsp pepper
- 2 tbs coconut oil
- 3/4 tsp thyme
- 1 tsp onion powder
- 3/4 tsp salt

- 2 cloves garlic
- 3/4 tsp garlic powder
- 1 2/3 cups coconut milk, full fat
- 3/4 tsp celery salt

Steps:

1. Pulse the cauliflower florets in a food blender for approximately 1 minute on high until crumbly.
2. Heat the cauliflower in a saucepan.
3. Scoop the cauliflower into a tea towel and twist to remove the moisture, repeating as necessary until as much of the water is removed as possible.
4. Heat a large pot and melt the coconut oil.
5. Mince the garlic and pour into the hot pot to simmer for approximately 2 minutes.
6. Combine the ground turkey to the garlic and brown for about 7 minutes, stirring with a wooden scraper to break up the meat.
7. Blend the riced cauliflower, salt, thyme, garlic powder, celery salt, mustard, and pepper with the meat until combined.
8. Reduce the temperature and finally add the coconut milk. Simmer for approximately 6 additional minutes.
9. Serve hot and enjoy!

Variation Tips:

- If you continue to reduce the dish by half and it will

become thicker and can be served as a dip at your next party.

- Alternatively, you can use ground pork, lamb or beef with this recipe. You can also add other vegetables such as broccoli.
- Optional garnishes include bacon, cherry tomatoes, hot sauce or jalapenos.

SNACK RECIPES

Mashed Cauliflower

Missing potatoes? You will not anymore with this brilliant substitution which tastes so good; you will not be able to taste the difference.

Total Prep & Cooking Time: 25 minutes Level: Beginner

Makes: 4 Helpings

Protein: 4 grams Net Carbs: 6 grams Fat: 13 grams

Sugar: 0 grams

Calories: 227

What you need:

- 1/2 cup chives, chopped
- 3 cups cauliflower
- 1 tsp salt
- 2 tbs olive oil
- 1/4 cup parsley
- 3 cloves garlic, chopped
- 1 tsp pepper
- 8 oz. sour cream
- 6 cups of water

Steps:

1. Boil the water in a large pot and sauté the cauliflower for approximately 15 minutes.
2. In a large dish, blend the chives, salt, olive oil, parsley, garlic, pepper, and sour cream until combined.
3. Drain the hot water from the cauliflower and crush completely until the consistency is smooth.
4. Integrate the mixture to the cauliflower, totally blending.
5. Wait about 5 minutes before serving.

Herb Bread

Serves: 4

Ingredients:

- 2 Tbsp Coconut Flour
- 1 ½ cups Almond Flour
- 2 Tbsp Fresh Herbs of choice, chopped
- 2 Tbsp Ground Flax Seeds
- 1 ½ tsp Baking Soda
- ¼ tsp Salt
- 5 Eggs
- 1 Tbsp Apple Cider Vinegar
- ¼ cup Coconut Oil, melted

Directions:

1. Preheat your oven to 350F / 175C. Grease a loaf pan and set aside.
2. Add the coconut flour, almond flour, herbs, flax, baking soda, and salt to your food processor. Pulse to combine and then add the eggs, vinegar, and oil.
3. Transfer the batter to the prepared loaf pan and bake in the preheated oven for about 30 min.

4. Once baked and golden brown, remove from the oven, set aside to cool, slice and eat.

Nutritional Values:

Calories: 421,

Total Fat: 37.4 g, Saturated Fat: 14.8 g, Carbs: 9.4 g, Sugars: 0.9 g, Protein: 15.1 g

Almond Bread

Serves: 8

Nutritional Values:

Calories: 277,

Total Fat: 21.5 g, Saturated Fat: 7.3 g, Carbs: 12.7 g,

Sugars: 0.3 g, Protein: 10.7 g

Ingredients:

- 1 1/4 cups Almond Flour
- 1/2 cup Coconut Flour
- 1/4 cup Ground Chia Seeds
- 1/2 tsp Baking Soda
- 1/4 tsp Salt
- 4 Tbsp Coconut Oil, melted
- 5 Eggs
- 1 Tbsp Apple Cider Vinegar

Directions:

1. Preheat your oven to 350F / 190C. Grease a loaf pan and set aside.
2. Combine all the dry ingredients and set aside.
3. Mix together the wet ingredients and add them to the dry ingredients. Mix well to combine.
4. Transfer the batter to the prepared loaf pan and bake in the preheated oven for about 40-50 minutes.
5. When baked, allow to cool, slice and eat.

Almond Keto Bread

Ingredients:

- 3 cups Almond Flour
- 1 tsp Baking Soda
- 2 tsp Baking Powder
- ¼ tsp Salt

¼ cup Almond Milk

- ½ cup + 2 Tbsp Olive Oil
- 3 Eggs

Serves: 10 slices **Nutritional**

Values: Calories: 302,

Total Fat: 28.6 g, Saturated Fat: 3 g,

Carbs: 7.3g,

Sugars: 1.2 g,

Protein: 8.5 g

Directions:

1. Preheat your oven to 300F / 149C. Grease a loaf pan (e.g. 9x5) and set aside.
2. Combine all the ingredients and transfer the batter to the prepared loaf pan.
3. Bake in the preheated oven for an hour.
4. Once baked, remove from the oven, allow to cool, slice and eat.

Thanksgiving Bread

Ingredients:

- 1 Tbsp Ghee
- 2 Celery Stalks, chopped
- 1 Onion, chopped
- ½ cup Walnuts
- ½ cup Coconut Flour
- 1½ cup Almond Flour
- 1 Tbsp Fresh Rosemary, chopped
- 10 Sage Leaves, finely chopped
- 1 tsp Baking Soda
- 1 pinch Freshly Grated Nutmeg
- ¼ tsp Salt½ cup Chicken Broth
- 4 Eggs
- 2-3 Bacon Strips, cooked and crumbled

Serves: 4

Nutritional Values:

Calories: 339, Total Fat: 26.9 g, Protein: 12.2 g`
Saturated Fat: 5.7 g, Carbs: 16.7 g,

Sugars: 1.2 g,

Directions:

1. Preheat your oven to 350F / 175C.

2. Add the ghee to a pan and melt on medium. Add the celery and onion and sauté for about 5 minutes.

3. Once tender, add the walnuts and cook for a few more minutes. Set aside.

4. In a bowl, mix together the coconut flour, almond flour, rosemary, sage, baking soda, nutmeg, and salt.

5. Mix in the sautéed celery and onion and add the chicken broth and eggs. Mix until well incorporated.

6. Stir in the bacon crumbles and transfer the batter to the prepared loaf pan. Bake n the preheated oven for about 30-35 minutes.

7. Once baked, leave to cool, slice and serve.

DINNER RECIPES

Chili Lime Drumsticks

Sink your teeth into this wonderful dinner that may just become your favorite flavorful meat on the Keto diet.

Total Prep & Cooking Time: 45 minutes plus 1 hour to marinate

Level: Beginner

Makes: 4 Helpings

Protein: 24 grams

Net Carbs: 1 gram Fat: 15 grams

Sugar: 0 grams

Calories: 249

What you need:

- 1 tsp chili powder
- 4 chicken drumsticks
- 2 tsp lime juice
- 1 tsp garlic powder
- 3 tsp avocado oil
- 1/4 tsp salt

Steps:

1. In a big lidded tub, blend the chili powder, avocado oil, garlic powder, and lime juice until incorporated.
2. Place the meat into the liquid and arrange to cover completely.
3. Marinate for at least 60 minutes or overnight.
4. When you are ready to cook, adjust your grill to heat at 450° Fahrenheit.
5. Take away the chicken from the marinade and grill for about 35 minutes making sure to turn them over approximately every 5 minutes. Check the temperate with a meat thermometer until they reach 185° Fahrenheit.
6. Dust with salt and serve hot.

UNUSUAL DELICIOUS MEAL RECIPES

Salmon Tartare

This would be the Keto diet´s version of raw fish sushi in this mini fat bomb that will have you smacking your lips.

Total Prep & Cooking Time: 25 minutes plus 2 hours to marinate (optional)

Level: Intermediate

Makes: 4 Helpings

Protein: 28 grams Net Carbs: 1.8 grams

Fat: 40 grams

Sugar: 0 grams

Calories: 272

What you need:

- 16 oz. salmon fillet, skinless
- 5 oz. smoked salmon
- 1/4 tsp cayenne pepper
- 4 oz. mayonnaise, sugar-free
- 1/4 cup parsley, chopped
- 4 oz. extra virgin olive oil
- 2 tbs lime juice
- 1 tbs caper brine
- 2 tbs green olives, chopped

- 1/4 tsp pepper
- 2 tbs capers, chopped
- 1 tsp mustard, dijon

Steps:

1. Slice the smoked and fresh salmon into cubes about 1/4 inch wide and toss into a glass dish.
2. Blend the mayonnaise, cayenne pepper, chopped olives, pepper and mustard with the salmon until combined thoroughly.
3. Finally integrate the parsley, olive oil, lime juice, capers, and caper brine until incorporated fully.
4. Layer plastic wrap over the bowl and refrigerate for approximately 2 hours to marinate properly.
5. Remove the salmon from the fridge and section the fish into 4 servings.
6. Use a large circle cookie cutter to lightly push the salmon into a thick patty using a spoon.
7. Remove the cookie cutter and garnish with a splash of olive oil and serve.

Baking Tips:

1. It is necessary to acquire fresh fish since this is a raw dish. If there is any skin on the salmon, it needs to be removed prior to cutting.
2. Take care when cutting the fish into cubes. If you cut them too small, the tartare will be mushy.
3. The marinating is not ultra-important to the dish, but it does help the ingredients to meld into each other properly.

KETO DESSERTS RECIPES

Chocó Chip Bars

Serves: 24

Preparation time: 10 minutes Cooking time: 35 minutes

Ingredients:

- 1 cup walnuts, chopped
- 1 ½ tsp baking powder
- 1 cup unsweetened chocolate chips
- 1 cup almond flour
- ¼ cup coconut flour
- 1 ½ tsp vanilla
- 5 eggs
- ½ cup butter
- 8 oz cream cheese
- 2 cups erythritol
- Pinch of salt

Directions:

1. 350 F/ 180 C should be the target when preheating oven.
2. Line cookie sheet with parchment paper and set

aside.

3. Beat together butter, sweetener, vanilla, and cream cheese until smooth.
4. Add eggs and beat until well combined.
5. Add remaining ingredients and stir gently to combine.
6. The mixture should be transferred to the prepared cookie sheet and spread evenly.
7. Bake in preheated oven for 35 minutes.
8. Remove from oven and allow to cool completely.
9. Slice and serve.

Per Serving: Net Carbs: 2.6g; Calories: 207 Total Fat: 18.8 g; Saturated Fat: 8.5g

Protein: 5.5g; Carbs: 4.8g; Fiber: 2.2g; Sugar: 0.4g; Fat 83% / Protein 11% / Carbs 6%

Sesame Bars

Serves: 16

Preparation time: 10 minutes Cooking time: 15 minutes

Ingredients:

- 1 1/4 cups sesame seeds
- 10 drops liquid stevia
- 1/2 tsp vanilla
- 1/4 cup unsweetened applesauce
- 3/4 cup coconut butter
- Pinch of salt

Directions:

1. Preheat the oven to 350 F/ 180 C.
2. Spray a baking dish with cooking spray and set aside.
3. In a large bowl, add applesauce, coconut butter, vanilla, liquid stevia, and sea salt and stir until well combined.
4. Add sesame seeds and stir to coat.
5. Pour mixture into a prepared baking dish and bake in preheated oven for 10-15 minutes.
6. Remove from oven and set aside to cool completely.
7. Place in refrigerator for 1 hour.
8. Cut into pieces and serve.

Per Serving: Net Carbs: 2.4g; Calories: 136 Total Fat: 12.4g; Saturated Fat: 6.8g

Protein: 2.8g; Carbs: 5.7g; Fiber: 3.3g; Sugar: 1.2g; Fat 83% / Protein 9% / Carbs 8%

CAKE

Easy Lemon Pie

Serves: 8

Preparation time: 10 minutes Cooking time: 45 minutes

Ingredients:

- 3 eggs
- 3 lemon juice
- 1 lemon zest, grated

- 4 oz erythritol
- oz almond flour
- oz butter, melted
- Salt

Directions:

1. Preheat the oven to 350 F/ 180 C.
2. In a bowl, mix together butter, 1 oz sweetener, 3 oz almond flour, and salt.
3. Transfer the dough in a pie dish and spread evenly and bake for 20 minutes.
4. In a separate bowl, mix together eggs, lemon juice, lemon zest, remaining flour, sweetener, and salt.
5. Pour egg mixture on prepared crust and bake for 25 minutes more.
6. Allow to cool completely.
7. Slice and serve.

Per Serving: Net Carbs: 3.0g; Calories: 229; Total Fat: 21.5g; Saturated Fat: 7.7g

Protein: 6.5g; Carbs: 5.3g; Fiber: 2.3g; Sugar: 1.4g; Fat 84% / Protein 11% / Carbs 5%

Delicious Pumpkin Cream Pie

Serves: 10

Preparation time: 10 minutes Cooking time: 60 minutes

For crust:

- 1 tsp erythritol
- 8 tbsp butter
- 1 ¼ cup almond flour
- Pinch of salt
- For filling:
- 2 eggs
- ½ tsp liquid stevia
- ½ cup erythritol
- 2 tbsp pumpkin pie spice
- ¼ cup sour cream
- ¾ cup heavy cream
- 15 oz can pumpkin puree

Directions:

1. For the crust: Preheat the oven to 350 F/ 180 C.
2. Add all crust ingredients into the food processor and process until dough is formed.
3. Transfer the dough in a pie dish and spread evenly.
4. Prick bottom on crust using fork or knife.
5. Bake crust in preheated oven for 10 minutes.

6. For the filling: Preheat the oven to 375 F/ 190 C.
7. In a large bowl, whisk eggs with sour cream, heavy cream, and pumpkin puree.
8. Add stevia, erythritol, and pumpkin pie spice and whisk well.
9. Pour cream pumpkin mixture into the baked crust and spread evenly.
10. Bake in preheated oven for 45-50 minutes.
11. Allow to cool completely then place in the refrigerator for 2-3 hours.
12. Serve and enjoy.

Per Serving: Net Carbs: 5.6g; Calories: 239; Total Fat: 21.8g; Saturated Fat: 9.5g

Protein: 5.3g; Carbs: 8.3g; Fiber: 2.7g; Sugar: 2.1g; Fat 83% / Protein 8% / Carbs 9%

CANDY: BEGINNER

Easy Peanut Butter Cookies

Serves: 15

Preparation time: 10 minutes Cooking time: 15 minutes

Ingredients:

- 1 egg
- ½ cup erythritol
- 1 cup peanut butter
- 1 tsp vanilla
- Pinch of salt

Directions:

1. Preheat the oven to 350 F/ 180 C.
2. Add all ingredients into the large bowl and mix until well combined.
3. Make cookies from bowl mixture and place on a baking tray.
4. Bake in preheated oven for 10-12 minutes.
5. Let it cool completely then serve.

Per Serving: Net Carbs: 2.5g; Calories: 106; Total Fat: 8.9g;

Saturated Fat: 1.9g

Protein: 4.7g; Carbs: 3.5g; Fiber: 1g; Sugar: 1.7g; Fat 75% /

Protein 17% / Carbs 8%

FROZEN DESSERT: BEGINNER

Expert: Classic Citrus Custard

Serves: 4

Preparation time: 10 minutes Cooking time: 10 minutes

Ingredients:

- 2 ½ cups heavy whipping cream
- ½ tsp orange extract
- 2 tbsp fresh lime juice
- ¼ cup fresh lemon juice
- ½ cup Swerve
- Pinch of salt

Directions:

1. Boil heavy whipping cream and sweetener in a saucepan for 5-6

minutes. Stir continuously.

2. Remove saucepan from heat and add orange extract, lime juice, lemon juice, and salt and mix well.
3. Pour custard mixture into ramekins.
4. Place ramekins in refrigerator for 6 hours.
5. Serve chilled and enjoy.

Per Serving: Net Carbs: 2.7g; Calories: 265; Total Fat: 27.9g; Saturated Fat: 17.4g

Protein: 1.7g; Carbs: 2.8g; Fiber: 0.1g; Sugar: 0.5g; Fat 94% / Protein 2% / Carbs 4%

BREAKFAST RECIPES

Keto Bacon and Split Pea Burgers

Absolute: 2 hr 20 min

Prep: 35 min

Dormant: 30 min

Cook: 1 hr 15 min

Yield: 8 (5-ounce) burgers

Ingredients

- 1 teaspoon ground coriander
- 1 tablespoon olive oil, in addition to 1 to 2 extra tablespoons for sauteing
- 1/2 cup cleaved onion
- 3 cups vegetable stock
- 1/2 cup cleaved chime pepper
- Genuine salt and newly ground dark pepper
- 2 teaspoons minced garlic
- 4 ounces mushrooms, cut
- 1/2 cup dry dark colored rice
- 1 teaspoon ground cumin
- 3/4 cup plain dry bread scraps, in addition to 1/4 cup for covering
- 1 cup dry split peas, picked and washed

Direction

1. Warmth 1 tablespoon olive oil in a huge (4 to 6-quart) pot over medium warmth. Include the onion and chime pepper alongside a liberal squeeze of salt. For 5 minutes sweat or until the onions are delicate. Include the garlic and mushrooms and keep on cooking for an additional 4 minutes.
2. Include the soup, peas, rice, coriander and cumin. Increment the warmth to high and heat to the point of boiling. Abatement warmth to low, spread and cook at a stew for 1 hour or until the rice and peas are delicate.
3. Expel from the warmth and tenderly empty the blend into the bowl of a nourishment processor and procedure until just combined.* Do not puree.

   Empty this blend into a bowl and mix in the 3/4 cup of bread morsels. Refrigerate for 30 minutes.
4. Shape the blend into patties and dig on each side in the rest of the 1/4 cup of bread morsels. Warm 1 tablespoon of olive oil in a medium saute container over medium warmth. Include 2 burgers at any given moment and saute until dark colored on each side, roughly 3 to 4 minutes for every side. To flame broil, cook on high for 3 to 4 minutes for each side also. Serve right away.

LUNCH RECIPES

Keto Strawberry Muffins

Cooking time: 20 min Yield: 12 muffins

Nutrition facts: 87 calories per muffin: Carbs 4.3g, fats 7g, and proteins 2.4g.

Ingredients:

- 10,5 oz almond flour
- 2 tsp baking powder
- 1/4 tsp salt
- 1 tsp cinnamon
- 8 tbsp sweetener
- 5 tbsp butter, melted
- 3 eggs
- 1 tsp vanilla extract
- 6 tbsp heavy cream
- 2/3 cup fresh strawberries

Steps:

1. Heat the oven to 175 C.
2. Beat together: melted butter+sweetener.
3. Add there: eggs+vanilla+cream. Go on beating until the dough is foamy.
4. Mix some sweetener with strawberries and put aside.

5. Sift together: almond flour+baking powder+salt+cinnamon.
6. Add the dry ingredients to the butter and eggs. Mix well.
7. Mix in strawberries.
8. Place the dough into the baking cups, greased.
9. Bake for 20 min.

SNACKS RECIPES

Garlic Breadsticks

Servings:8 breadsticks

Nutritional Values: Calories: 259.2, Total Fat: 24.7 g, Saturated Fat: 7.5 g, Carbs: 6.3 g, Sugars: 1.1 g, Protein: 7 g

Ingredients for the garlic butter:

- 1/4 cup Butter, softened
- 1 tsp Garlic Powder
- Ingredients:
- 2 cup Almond Flour
- 1/2 Tbsp Baking Powder
- 1 Tbsp Psyllium Husk Powder
- 1/4 tsp Salt
- 3 Tbsp Butter, melted
- 1 Egg
- 1/4 cup Boiling Water

Directions:

1. Preheat your oven to 400F / 200C.
2. Beat the garlic powder and butter and set aside to use it for brushing.
3. Combine the psyllium husk powder,

   baking powder, almond flour and salt. Add the butter along with the egg and mix until well combined.
4. Mix until dough forms using boiling water.
5. Divide into breadsticks.
6. Bake for 15 minutes. Brush the breadsticks with the garlic butter and bake for 5 more minutes.

Serve warm or allow to cool.

Savory Italian Crackers

Servings:20-30 crackers

Nutritional Values: Calories: 63.5, Total Fat: 5.8 g, Saturated Fat: 0.6 g, Carbs: 1.8 g, Sugars: 0.3 g, Protein: 2.1 g

Ingredients:

- 1 1/2 cup Almond Flour
- 1/4 tsp Garlic Powder
- 1/2 tsp Onion Powder
- 1/2 tsp Thyme
- 1/4 tsp Basil
- 1/4 tsp Oregano
- 3/4 tsp Salt
- 1 Egg
- 2 Tbsp Olive Oil

Directions:

1. Preheat your oven to 350F / 175C.
2. Combine until dough forms.
3. Form a log and slice into thin crackers. Arrange the crackers onto the prepared baking sheet and bake for about 10-15 minutes.
4. When done, allow to cool and serve.

THE KETO LUNCH

Saturday: Lunch: Chicken Noodle-less Soup

All the comfort of a classic soup without the carbs. How comforting.

Variation tip: use the meat from a rotisserie chicken.

Prep Time: 10 minutes Cook Time: 20 minutes Serves 4

What's in it

- Butter (.25 cup)
- Celery (1 stalk)
- Mushrooms (3 ounces)
- Garlic, minced (1 clove)
- Dried minced onion (1 T)
- Dried parsley (1 t)
- Chicken stock (4 cups)
- Kosher salt (.5 t)
- Fresh ground pepper (.25 t)
- Carrot, chopped (1 qty)
- Chicken, cooked and diced (2.5 cups or 1.5 pounds of

chicken breast)

- Cabbage, sliced (1 cups)

How it's made

Put large soup pot on medium heat and melt butter.

Slice the celery and mushrooms and add, along with dried onion to the pot.

Add parsley, broth, carrot, kosher salt and fresh pepper. Stir.

Simmer until veggies are tender.

Stir in cooked chicken and sliced cabbage. Simmer until cabbage is tender, about 8 to 12 minutes.

Net carbs: 4 grams Fat: 40 grams

Protein: 33 grams

Sugars: 1 gram

KETO AT DINNER

Saturday: Dinner:

"Breaded" Pork Chops

With crispy, keto friendly breading, this is sure to be a family favorite.

Variation tip: if you can spare the calories, sprinkle with shredded Parmesan cheese.

Prep Time: 5 minutes Cook Time: 30 minutes

Serves 4

What's in it

- Boneless thin pork chops (4 qty)
- Psyllium husk powder (1 T)
- Kosher salt (.5 t)
- Paprika (.25 t)
- Garlic powder (.25 t)
- Onion powder (.25 t)
- Oregano (.25 t)

How it's made

1. Preheat oven to 350 degrees F.
2. Dry pork chops with a paper towel.
3. Combine the rest of the ingredients in a ziplock bag.

4. One at a time, seal the pork chops in the bag and shake to coat.
5. Put a wire rack on a baking sheet. Place pork chops on rack.
6. Bake in oven for approximately 30 minutes. The thermometer should read 145 degrees F.
7. Serve with vegetables or a green salad.

Net carbs: 0 grams

Fat: 9 grams

Protein: 28 grams

Sugars: 0 grams

CPSIA information can be obtained
at www.ICGtesting.com
Printed in the USA
BVHW062031020321
601494BV00010B/844

9 781801 949187